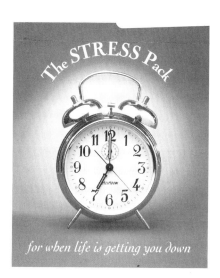

The STRESS Pack

for when life is getting you down

CHRISTINE FALVEY

Contents

Contents

*My life is one
demd horid grind!*

Charles Dickens — *Nicholas Nickleby*

INTRODUCTION

These days it can seem that the whole world finds life one demd horid grind with the word "stress" a regular in everyone's vocabulary. If we're not just plain stressed, we're under stress, suffering from stress or "stressed-out".

Some of us feel silently anxious about everything and nothing all the time. Others constantly feel jumpy and irritable, ready either to burst into tears or a rage. Stress can send us into a dithery panic, or virtually immobilise us. One way or another, stress seems to have reduced our sense of the joy of life to a grinding, debilitating strain.

Stress though, is a necessary part of life. Imagine life without the joyful stress of learning to walk or swim or read, of succeeding in your new job or promotion or of being in love.

This book invites you to free yourself of excess stress by presenting dozens of tips and techniques all geared to helping you to avoid the harmful stresses that come your way and to improve your ability to cope with those unavoidable ones.

But if you were never stressed, you'd never know what it was to be alive. To eliminate your capacity to experience stress would be to eliminate the excitement of a new love affair, a forthcoming party, a new job or promotion, indeed any situation which involves decisions, hopes and desires.

*Stress can be a wild thing —
it needs to be controlled rather than tamed.
It is negative stress, uncontrolled stress,
that is dangerous to your mental and physical health.
When it becomes a pattern of life, you are in trouble.*

The aim of this book is to offer you ways of eliminating unnecessary stress while simultaneously improving your ability to deal with it.

Discover just how easy — and how much fun — it can be to get your stress under control and in its right perspective.

I love living. I have some problems with my life, but living is the best thing they've come up with so far.

Neil Simon — *Last of the Red Hot Lovers*

STRESS AT WORK

Time management

ARE YOU ALWAYS RACING THE CLOCK? ALWAYS RUNNING LATE?

REVIEW YOUR PLANNING. ARE YOU ALLOWING ENOUGH TIME TO PLAN THINGS AS WELL AS DO THEM?

DO ALL YOU CAN TO ENSURE THINGS GO AS PLANNED. ESTABLISH WHAT MATTERS, ELIMINATE ELEMENTS THAT ARE NOT NECESSARY TO THE SITUATION, THEN TRY AND IDENTIFY WEAK OR DIFFICULT AREAS IN ADVANCE SO YOU CAN PLAN COMPENSATORY ACTION IF NEEDED.

YOU CAN NEVER COMPLETELY ELIMINATE SURPRISES, BUT AT LEAST THIS WAY YOU'LL BE WELL-PREPARED AND IN A POSITION TO KNOW WHAT YOU CAN CHANGE — AND WHAT YOU CAN'T.

Managing stress the 21st century way

*NOW YOU CAN BUY COMPUTER SOFTWARE
DESIGNED TO HELP YOU RELAX.*

ONE PACKAGE WORKS USING ELECTRODES CONNECTED TO YOUR FINGERS. THE DATA GATHERED IS FED TO YOUR PERSONAL COMPUTER BY A CORDLESS, INFRA-RED LINK. THE FEEDBACK IS CONVERTED TO GRAPHICS SYMBOLIZING YOUR DEGREE OF STRESS OR RELAXATION.

ANOTHER MEASURES THE USER'S RESPONSES TO MUSIC, VOICES AND SUNDRY IMAGES, THEN DISPENSES ADVICE ON RELAXATION TECHNIQUES APPROPRIATE TO THE LEVEL OF STRESS IT HAS ANALYSED.

OR YOU MIGHT OPT FOR THE PACKAGE THAT DELIVERS THE USER WITH AN ANALYSIS OF HIS OR HER STRESS LEVEL, STRESS SOURCES, A STRESS PROFILE AND A PERSONAL STRESS MANAGEMENT PLAN.

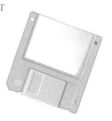

Nothing energises an individual ...
more than clear goals and a grand
purpose. Nothing demoralises
more than confusion ....

Tony O'Reilly — CEO of H.J. Heinz

Goals

A GOAL THAT IS NOT ONE YOU TRULY CARE ABOUT YOURSELF BUT IS ONE FORMULATED TO GAIN ACCEPTANCE OR APPROVAL OF ONE KIND OR ANOTHER IS A MAJOR CAUSE OF STRESS.

MAKE A LIST OF YOUR GOALS. THEN PUT THEM INTO ORDER OF PRIORITY.

WOULD YOU STAND A BETTER CHANCE OF SUCCESS, A BETTER CHANCE OF ACHIEVING YOUR GOALS, IF YOU MANAGED YOUR STRESS RESPONSES BETTER? IF THE ANSWER IS "YES", PUT BETTER STRESS MANAGEMENT RIGHT AT THE TOP OF YOUR LIST.

SORT EACH OF YOUR GOALS INTO ITS COMPONENTS. DECIDE WHAT YOU NEED TO DO TO REALIZE EACH ONE. SET YOURSELF A SCHEDULE FOR ACHIEVEMENT.

Test your goals

DISCUSS THEM WITH YOUR MENTOR,
YOUR FRIENDS, YOUR FAMILY.

ARE YOU PREPARED TO FORGO SOME OF YOUR CURRENT ACTIVITIES OR INTERESTS IN ORDER TO FULFIL THEM?

WHAT CAN YOU DELEGATE? DO YOU FIND IT DIFFICULT TO DELEGATE? PERHAPS YOU NEED TO PRACTICE DELEGATING — SMALL TASKS WILL DO TO BEGIN WITH.

AND PRACTICE SAYING "NO". THIS IS VERY DIFFICULT FOR SOME PEOPLE SO AGAIN BEGIN IN A SMALL WAY. YOU WILL BE SURPRISED HOW THE OTHER PERSON ACCEPTS WITHOUT QUESTION YOUR LACK OF AVAILABILITY TO HELP IN THAT PARTICULAR MATTER; THEY WILL GO AND FIND SOMEBODY ELSE. SOON, PEOPLE WILL STOP AUTOMATICALLY SEEING YOU AS THEIR OWN PERSONAL PROBLEM-SOLVER AND YOU WILL HAVE LOST NO FRIENDS.

EXERCISE

Stress has gotten a bad name. Stress of all kinds is good — physical, emotional and mental. It's strengthening. What troubles us is the absence of recovery strategies needed to balance the stress.

James Loehr — sports psychologist

STOMACH CRUNCHES ARE HIGH ON JAMES LOEHR'S LIST OF STRESSBUSTERS. THESE MINI SIT-UPS WORK WONDERS ON YOUR ABDOMINAL MUSCLES, THOSE CRUCIAL SUPPORTS WHICH HELP YOU STAND TALL, BREATHE DEEPER, FEEL BETTER.

LIE ON THE FLOOR ON YOUR BACK, KNEES BENT, ARMS AT YOUR SIDES, CHIN GENTLY TUCKED. NOW LIFT YOUR SHOULDERS ABOUT 5 CM FROM THE FLOOR. THIS EXERCISE IS A LOT EASIER THAN SIT-UPS. DO THIS 100 TIMES IF YOU CAN, OTHERWISE DO SAY 20 THEN EACH TIME BUILD ON ANOTHER 10 UNTIL YOU REACH THE GOAL OF 100. FIVE MINUTES LATER YOU'LL WALK TALL AND FEEL THAT YOU CAN CARRY ALL BEFORE YOU.

*It is a good morning exercise
for a research scientist to discard
a pet hypothesis every day
before breakfast.*

Konrad Lorenz — *On Aggression*

AROMATHERAPY

Scent to de-stress

AROMATHERAPY IS A GREAT WAY TO LOOK AFTER YOURSELF, PAMPER YOURSELF. SHOW YOURSELF YOU CARE — ABOUT YOU. IT WILL PUT YOU IN TOUCH WITH YOUR SENSES — ONE OF THE FIRST ASPECTS OF YOURSELF YOU LOSE WHEN YOU'RE SUFFERING STRESS.

TAKE AN AROMATIC BATH. SOAK YOUR FEET IN A FOOTBATH IF YOUR BATHROOM DOESN'T POSSESS A BATHTUB. GIVE YOURSELF A MASSAGE. LOUNGE ABOUT IN A ROOM SCENTED WITH AN ESSENTIAL OIL THAT APPEALS TO YOU. SPRINKLE IT ON YOUR FAVORITE CUSHIONS AND THROW-OVERS WHEN CURLED UP IN RELAXING MODE. USE ESSENTIAL OILS AS PERFUME TO PLEASE YOU. A LITTLE DAB WILL HELP YOU FORGET YOUR STRESS.

CHANCES ARE THAT SPOILING YOURSELF WILL BE A LUXURY YOU'VE NOT ALLOWED YOURSELF IN ANY SHAPE OR FORM FOR A LONG, LONG TIME. THE BONUS IS THAT THESE AROMATIC OILS TRULY MAKE YOU FEEL BETTER. THEY ARE HEALING. AND YOU CAN HAVE FUN IN THE PROCESS.

THINK ABOUT IT. BATHING MEANS YOU GET TO PLAY WITH WATER, A NATURAL, SENSUAL, RELAXING EXPERIENCE IN ITSELF. AND WHO WILL KNOW IF YOU SPLASH AROUND WITH A LITTLE YELLOW DUCK? BUT PERHAPS YOU'D PREFER TO LEAN BACK LANGUIDLY BY CANDLELIGHT WITH BACH OR BEETHOVEN, FLOATING YOUR ARMS AND LEGS, WHILE SWIRLING YOUR FINGERS THROUGH THE WATER.

SCIENTIFICALLY SPEAKING, THIS IS CALLED A COMPOUND EFFECT. TRANSLATION: DOUBLE OR TRIPLE WHAMMY TO OUR ENEMY WITHIN: STRESS.

BEFORE TURNING ON THE WARM TAP WATER, YOU CAN TAKE YOUR TIME LUXURIATING IN PICKING WHICH OF THE MANY ESSENTIAL OILS IS THE ONE OR MORE FOR YOU.

ESSENTIAL OILS EVAPORATE VERY QUICKLY FROM THE LARGE SURFACE OF A BATHTUB FULL OF VERY HOT WATER, SO THINK OF WARM RATHER THAN HOT WATER BATHS. A FEW DROPS OF OIL UPON THE SURFACE, WHISKED LIGHTLY WITH YOUR FINGERTIPS TO FORM A FILM THERE, WILL COAT YOUR SKIN AS YOU SUBMERGE YOUR — YOU WILL NOTICE — QUITE RIGID BODY. FIFTEEN MINUTES OF SIMULTANEOUS SOAKING AND INHALATION OF YOUR FRAGRANT BATH IS USUALLY LONG ENOUGH TO DO THE TRICK.

Make a full-body massage oil by combining a total of 25 drops of essential oil or oils to 2 fl oz (50 ml) of a carrier oil. Cold-pressed vegetable oils such as sweet almond, apricot kernel, grapeseed, avocado and jojoba make the best carrier oils. For smaller quantities, sufficient to give a stress-relieving massage to parts of the body such as the feet or face, add 6 to 9 drops of essential oil to 1/2 fl oz (15 ml) of carrier oil or 3 to 6 drops of essential oil to 1 teaspoon (5 ml) of carrier oil.

AMONG THOSE ESSENTIAL OILS WIDELY RECOGNIZED AS ANTI-STRESS IN EFFECT ARE BERGAMOT, CHAMOMILE, CLARY SAGE, CYPRESS, FRANKINCENSE, GERANIUM, JUNIPER, LAVENDER, MARJORAM, ORANGE BLOSSOM, PATCHOULI, ROSE, SANDALWOOD, AND YLANG-YLANG.

SUPERMARKETS, PHARMACIES AND NATURAL LIFESTYLE BOUTIQUES ARE GOOD SOURCES OF A WIDE RANGE OF AROMATHERAPY OILS AND EQUIPMENT INCLUDING VAPORIZERS AND SUITABLE SPRAY BOTTLES AND CARRIER OILS.

ONE OF THE MOST DIRECT WAYS TO EXPERIENCE AN AROMATHERAPEUTIC EFFECT IS THROUGH A STEAM INHALATION. NO SPECIAL EQUIPMENT IS REQUIRED. JUST A KITCHEN BOWL OR BASIN TO WHICH YOU ADD UP TO 10 DROPS OF YOUR CHOSEN ESSENTIAL OIL AND BOILING WATER. DRAPE A TOWEL OVER YOUR HEAD AND NECK TO FORM A LITTLE STEAM TENT, BEND YOUR FACE OVER THE BOWL AND INHALE GENTLY.

LAVENDER (*LAVANDULA OFFICINALIS*) ACTS LIKE A HEAT-SEEKING MISSILE WHEN STRESS IS ABOUT. A SNIFF OR TWO FROM YOU AND LAVENDER WILL SEARCH AND DESTROY THE MONSTER. USE IT ALONE OR TEAM IT UP WITH ALMOST ANY OTHER ESSENTIAL OIL YOU FANCY. IT WORKS PARTICULARLY WELL WITH CHAMOMILE, FRANKINCENSE, GERANIUM, JUNIPER, MARJORAM, ORANGE BLOSSOM AND YLANG YLANG.

BERGAMOT (*CITRUS BERGAMIA*) GOES ESPECIALLY WELL WITH LAVENDER AND YOU CAN ALSO MIX IT ALONE OR WITH LAVENDER TO MAKE A THREESOME WITH EITHER CHAMOMILE, CYPRESS, FRANKINCENSE, JUNIPER, MARJORAM, ORANGE BLOSSOM, PATCHOULI OR YLANG YLANG.

CHAMOMILE (*CHAMAEMELUM NOBILE, ANTHEMIS NOBILIS, MATRICARIA RECUTITA, MATRICARIA CHAMOMILLA*), LAVENDER-LOVER THAT IT IS, IS ALSO THE BEST OF FRIENDS WITH PATCHOULI AND ROSE AS WELL AS TEAMING BEAUTIFULLY WITH BERGAMOT.

CLARY SAGE (*Salvia sclarea*) PARTNERS BERGAMOT, CYPRESS, JUNIPER, ORANGE BLOSSOM AND ROSE.

CEDARWOOD (*Juniperus virginiana*) HAS AN EXHILARATING SCENT TO LIFT FLAGGING SPIRITS AND ALSO CALMS FRAZZLED NERVES.

FRANKINCENSE (*Boswellia carteri*) IS ANOTHER ESSENTIAL OIL WITH A SPECIAL AFFINITY WITH LAVENDER. REVEL IN THEIR COMPATIBILITY BUT DON'T DENY YOURSELF THE PLEASURE OF EXPERIMENTING WITH FRANKINCENSE AND BERGAMOT, ROSE OR SANDALWOOD.

GERANIUM (*Pelargonium graveolens*) IS AMAZINGLY COMPATIBLE WITH LAVENDER AND ALMOST ANY OTHER ESSENTIAL OIL. THREE ESSENTIAL OILS WHICH COMBINE WELL WITH GERANIUM (WITH OR WITHOUT LAVENDER) ARE BERGAMOT, JUNIPER OR PATCHOULI.

JUNIPER (*JUNIPERIS COMMUNIS*) AND LAVENDER ALONE ARE A GREAT ANTI-STRESS COMBINATION AS ARE JUNIPER-GERANIUM OR JUNIPER-BERGAMOT BLENDS.

MARJORAM (*ORIGANUM MARJORANA*), WORKS BETTER WITH LAVENDER THAN WITH ANY OTHER ESSENTIAL OIL TO DEFUSE THAT TICKING STRESS-BOMB, RELIEVE INSOMNIA, OR TO GENTLY REASSEMBLE YOURSELF IF YOUR PSYCHE FEELS ALREADY SHATTERED.

ORANGE BLOSSOM OIL (*CITRUS AURANTIUM*) WILL RELIEVE ANXIETY, STRESS-INDUCED DEPRESSION AND INSOMNIA. ITS SOOTHING, CALMING AND RELAXING PROPERTIES DISPEL PANIC. IT BLENDS SUPERBLY WITH LAVENDER, BERGAMOT OR CLARY SAGE IN AN ATOMIZER OR WHEN ADDED TO A BATH.

PATCHOULI (*POGOSTEMON PATCHOULI*) IS AS PERFECT WITH ROSE AS IT IS WITH BERGAMOT, CHAMOMILE OR GERANIUM OR YLANG YLANG. ADD LAVENDER AS A THIRD OIL OR USE WITH LAVENDER ALONE.

ROSE (*ROSA DAMASCENA*) IS SECOND ONLY TO LAVENDER IN ITS COMPATIBILITY WITH MOST OTHER ESSENTIAL OILS. WHEN STRESS REACHES HORROR LEVELS, CONSIDER MIXING ROSE WITH CLARY SAGE OR SANDALWOOD, CHAMOMILE, FRANKINCENSE AND PATCHOULI.

SANDALWOOD (*SANTALUM ALBUM*) LIKES YLANG YLANG AS WELL AS CYPRESS, FRANKINCENSE AND ROSE.

YLANG YLANG (*CANANGA ODORATA*) MINGLES WELL WITH PATCHOULI ALONE, WITH BERGAMOT OR SANDALWOOD, OR BERGAMOT AND SANDALWOOD TOGETHER.

... There's no need to worry -
Whatever you do, life is hell.

Wendy Cope — *Advice to Young Women*

HERBAL RELAXERS

THERE ARE DOZENS OF HERBAL REMEDIES WHICH PROMOTE BOTH A RELAXED MIND AND A RELAXED BODY. MANY OF THEM INCLUDE THE FOLLOWING HERBS IN THEIR LISTS OF INGREDIENTS: CATMINT, CHAMOMILE, GINSENG, HOREHOUND, LEMON BALM, LIMEFLOWER, PASSIONFLOWER, ROSEMARY, SCULLCAP, ST JOHN'S WORT, VERVAIN AND VALERIAN.

HERBAL TEAS ARE THE CLASSIC FORM OF REMEDY BUT COOKING WITH ANTI-STRESS HERBS IS ANOTHER EFFECTIVE AND CULINARILY CLEVER WAY TO INCORPORATE THEM IN YOUR DIET.

MANY HERBAL TEAS CAN NOW BE BOUGHT AS TEA BAGS. AS A RULE, YOU NEED 1 TEA BAG PER CUP OF TEA, BUT IF YOU'RE NEW TO HERBAL TEAS, YOU MIGHT FIND YOU NEED ONLY STEEP THE TEA BAG FOR A MINUTE OR TWO AT MOST, GRADUALLY STRENGTHENING THE TASTE BY STEEPING TO ABOUT 5 MINUTES.

If using dried herbs, use approximately ½ tablespoon of the dried leaves, petals or flower heads.

If using fresh flower heads, petals or leaves, you'll need about 1 tablespoon.

When the seeds or roots of herbs are used for tea, you generally need to let them steep for 5 to 10 minutes before straining.

CATMINT (*Nepeta cataria*) tea will calm your nerves, your muscles and at the same time ease the digestive disorders which often accompany excessive stress.

CHAMOMILE flowers, in cheerful colors of yellow and white, make a tea which eases feelings of restlessness and anxiety. Chamomile also relieves physical symptoms such as dyspepsia and various symptoms of tension reflected in a dysfunctioning digestive system such as nausea, heartburn or stomach discomfort.

CHAMOMILE TEA SWEETENED WITH HONEY WILL HELP CALM A DISTRESSED CHILD WHILE MANY WOMEN WHO SUFFER FROM PRE-MENSTRUAL TENSION SWEAR BY ITS CALMING PROPERTIES.

MANZANILLA SHERRY IS FLAVORED WITH CHAMOMILE, SO TRY A DROP BEFORE DINNER.

IN SUMMERTIME, WHEN HEAT SEEMS TO BE MAKING EVERYTHING WORSE, CHAMOMILE, AS CHILLED CHAMOMILE TEA OR AS CHAMOMILE COOLER, CAN HELP TAKE THE HEAT OUT OF EVERYTHING, INCLUDING STRESSFUL SITUATIONS AND STATES OF MIND.

CHAMOMILE COOLER

Steep about 10 sprigs of chamomile in 16 fl oz (500 ml)
of Manzanilla or medium-dry sherry for a couple of hours.
Then strain the sherry, adding to it another 16 fl oz (500 ml)
of chilled orange or apple juice.

AND IF YOU CAN FIND A CHAMOMILE LAWN TO LIE IN, OR A
CHAMOMILE COVERED GARDEN BENCH TO SIT ON, YOU'LL
FEEL VERY MUCH BETTER FOR INHALING ITS RELAXING
FRAGRANCE.

To comfort the braine, smel to camomill, ... sleep
reasonably, delight to heare melody and singing.

Ram's Little Dodoen (early seventeenth century)

AND AT THE END OF THE DAY, A LIGHT COTTON OR MUSLIN
SWAG OF CHAMOMILE LEAVES IN YOUR BATH WILL SOOTHE
AND REVIVE YOU AND HELP DISSIPATE STRESS.

THE FINELY GROUND ROOTS OF ALL THE **GINSENGS**, AMERICAN (*PANAX QUINQUEFOLIUM*), ASIATIC (*PANAX GINSENG*) AND SIBERIAN (*ELEUTHEROCOCCUS SENTICOCUS*) ARE RELAXANTS. AMERICAN GINSENG IS PARTICULARLY GOOD FOR DIGESTIVE SYMPTOMS OF STRESS. THE ASIATIC AND SIBERIAN GINSENGS ARE RENOWNED FOR THEIR PREVENTIVE QUALITIES IN PROMOTING GENERAL WELL-BEING, PARTICULARLY PHYSICAL STAMINA, AND ALSO FOR IMPROVING CONCENTRATION AND MENTAL ALERTNESS AT TIMES OF STRESS.

IF YOU KNOW THAT YOU'VE A STRESSFUL TIME AHEAD OF YOU, YOU MIGHT CONSIDER INCLUDING THESE GINSENGS IN YOUR DIET. GINSENGS THOUGH, ARE NOT RECOMMENDED FOR CHILDREN, FOR WOMEN EXPERIENCING MENSTRUAL STRESS, OR FOR ANYONE LONG TERM. AND IF YOU WANT TO TAKE ASIATIC OR SIBERIAN GINSENG, BE PREPARED TO GIVE UP YOUR CAFFEINE-LOADED TEA AND COFFEE. TO CONSUME EITHER OF THESE PLUS CAFFEINE WILL STIMULATE MORE PHYSICAL STRESS FOR YOUR BODY, NOT YOUR BODY'S CAPACITY TO COPE WITH IT.

FEELING TWITCHY AND STRUNG-OUT?

CHOOSE EITHER OF THE **HOREHOUNDS** — THE BLACK (*BALLOTA NIGRA*) OR THE WHITE (*MARRUBIUM VULGARE*) — TO MAKE TEA TO BE SIPPED SLOWLY TWO TO THREE TIMES DAILY. IF YOU FIND THE BITTER TASTE TOO MUCH, ADD HONEY TO TASTE.

FEEL YOUR CHEST RELAX, YOUR DIAPHRAGM, YOUR MID-BACK. FEEL YOURSELF BREATHING MORE EASILY, RELAXING.

> *Balm causeth the mind and the*
> *heart to become merry.*

Eleventh century Arabian healer, Avicenna.

THE MINTY, BRIGHT GREEN LEAVES AND TINY WHITE FLOWERS OF **LEMON BALM** (*MELISSA OFFICINALIS*) ARE MIXED TO PRODUCE A TEA WHICH CALMS THE CENTRAL NERVOUS SYSTEM AS WELL AS THE DIGESTIVE SYSTEM. WHEN A BUSY LIFE, OR JUST A PARTICULARLY BUSY DAY, HAS LEFT YOU OR YOUR CHILDREN FEELING UPTIGHT OR GENERALLY OUT OF SORTS, TRY A CUP OF LEMON BALM TEA TO SET THINGS RIGHT.

Baume drunke in wine ... comforts the heart, and driveth away all melancholy and sadnesse.

Late sixteenth century English herbalist,
John Gerard.

TOSS LEMON AND HONEY SCENTED LEMON BALM LEAVES INTO ALCOHOLIC AND NON-ALCOHOLIC FRUIT PUNCHES OR CITRUS TARTS. TRY IT WITH FISH INSTEAD OF ORDINARY LEMON. LEMON BALM AND/OR ROSEMARY LIFTS ROAST VEAL AND LAMB AS WELL AS YOUR SPIRITS. ANOTHER EXCELLENT DISH FOR STRESS IS VEAL WITH MUSHROOMS FLAVORED BY LEMON BALM.

A BATH TREATED WITH A HANDFUL EACH OF **LEMON BALM** AND **MARIGOLD** (*CALENDULA OFFICINALIS*) FLOWERS AND LEAVES WILL SOAK AWAY TENSION AND STRESS FROM TIRED LIMBS AND ACHING MUSCLES.

LIME FLOWER (*TILIA CORDATA* OR *PLATYPHYLLOS*) IS A GENTLE SOOTHER, ESPECIALLY GOOD AT NIGHTFALL, TAKEN AS TEA OR ADDED TO THE BATH WATER.

WHEN IT'S AGITATION, IRRITATION AND INAPPROPRIATE FURY THAT'S RAGING INSIDE YOU RATHER THAN PASSION OF A LOVING KIND, TRY TEA MADE WITH FLOWERS OF THE PASSION FRUIT VINE. **PASSIONFLOWER** (*PASSIFLORA INCARNATA*) TEA CAN BE TAKEN THROUGHOUT THE DAY AND BY BEDTIME YOU'LL BE SWEETLY RELAXED AND READY FOR A GOOD NIGHT'S SLEEP.

When angry, count four; when very angry, swear.
Mark Twain — *Pudd'nhead Wilson*

ROSEMARY (*ROSMARINUS OFFICINALIS*) IS A HERB THAT WILL PICK YOU UP WHEN STRESS HAS GOT YOU DOWN, DEPRESSED AND LETHARGIC. WHEN YOU'RE FEELING A MITE FLAKEY OR SHAKEY, YOUR STOMACH'S PLAYING UP WITH TENSION, AND YOU DON'T WANT TO THINK TOO MUCH ABOUT YOUR LIVER, ROSEMARY WILL GIVE YOU A LIFT. EVEN SNIFFING YOUR FINGERS AFTER RUBBING ROSEMARY WILL CLEAR YOUR HEAD AND TRIGGER A SURGE OF DELIGHT.

IT'S TRADITIONALLY USED TO FLAVOR LAMB, BUT ALSO USE IT TO FLAVOR PORK. ADD TENDER, YOUNG LEAVES TO BREAD DOUGHS AND TO FRESH SALADS. USE SPRIGS OF ROSEMARY TO FLAVOR OILS AND VINEGARS FOR DRESSINGS, HONEY FOR SWEETENERS.

ONE OF SCULLCAP'S COMMON NAMES IS MAD-DOG WEED BECAUSE EIGHTEENTH CENTURY EUROPEAN HEALERS BELIEVED IT TO BE A CURE FOR RABIES — HEREIN LIES A CLUE.

EITHER *SCUTELLARIA LATERIFOLIA* OR *SCUTELLARIA GALERICULATA* WILL CALM YOU DOWN SO THAT YOU NO LONGER FEEL SO AGGRESSIVE AND HOSTILE TO THE WORLD. INSTEAD YOU'LL FIND THAT END-OF-THE-TETHER FEELING DISSIPATING AS STRESS-EXHAUSTION IS ALLEVIATED AND YOUR ENERGY IS FREE ONCE MORE TO COPE WITH LIVING. SCULLCAP IS OFTEN RECOMMENDED TO EASE THE STRESS INVOLVED IN WEANING ONESELF OFF TOBACCO OR ALCOHOL.

STRESS

QUAINTLY NAMED IT MAY BE, BUT **ST JOHN'S WORT** (*HYPERICUM PERFORATUM*) IS A TONIC FOR TWENTIETH CENTURY NERVOUS SYSTEMS AFFLICTED BY ANXIETY, TENSION AND IRRITABILITY, AND FOR HEARTS AND MINDS BELEAGUERED BY THE BLUES AND THE WEARINESS THAT STRESS BRINGS IN ITS WAKE.

VERVAIN OR VERBENA (*VERBENA OFFICINALIS*) IS ANOTHER HERB KNOWN TO RESTORE CALM AND ENERGY IN PLACE OF NERVOUS EXHAUSTION. USE IT IN YOUR BATH FOR A SUPER-RELAXING EFFECT, COMBINING IT WITH LAVENDER TO REFRESH YOU.

THE HERB **VALERIAN** (*VALERIANA OFFICINALIS*), ONCE KNOWN AS ALL-HEAL, IS PARTICULARLY GOOD TO TAKE AT BEDTIME. IT CALMS WITHOUT SEDATING, ENABLING YOU TO ENTER A NATURAL, HEALTHY SLEEP — ONE OF THE BEST STRESS-RELIEVERS OF ALL. FOR A SOPHISTICATED NIGHTCAP, ADD 2 CUPS OF BOILING WATER TO 2 TEASPOONS OF VALERIAN, 1 TEASPOON OF GOOD CIDER VINEGAR, 3 TEASPOONS OF HONEY AND A DASH OF VODKA.

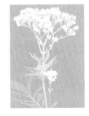

Massaging Away Stress

There's no better way than a massage to reduce distress. It reduces your stress to a level acceptable to you and those in your life who can be as much the casualties of your stress as you are. Consider co-opting one of your victims to engage in a mutual de-stressing massage or do it yourself. Set the scene by warming the room, use a vaporizer to scent it with your chosen essential oil, and after an aromatic bath, when your skin is warm and slightly damp, begin the massage.

A full body massage

START WITH THE FEET AND WORK YOUR WAY UP THE BODY: LOWER LEGS, AROUND THE KNEES, THE THIGHS, BUTTOCKS, ABDOMEN, MIDRIFF, BACK, SHOULDERS, NECK AND HEAD. STROKE EACH BODY PART FIRST WITH LIGHT, FEATHERY STROKES, THEN STRONGER ONES AND EVENTUALLY INTRODUCE A KNEADING, ROLLING MASSAGE ACTION. FOR THE ABDOMEN, MASSAGE GENTLY IN A CLOCKWISE DIRECTION. CONCLUDE THE MASSAGE WITH BUTTERFLY-BRUSHING, IMAGINING YOUR FINGERTIPS AS BUTTERFLY WINGS CARESSING YOU FROM HEAD DOWN TO YOUR TOES.

A facial massage

Bring your palms to meet in the middle of your face, fingertips resting on your forehead at your hairline. Make sweeping strokes outwards, working down your face and under your chin. Lean your head slightly to one side and with the backs of your hands and using a rolling, hand over hand movement, massage your neck with a series of quick strokes. Using the same technique, stimulate your face from jaw to cheekbone. Repeat the process for the opposite side of your neck and face before moving on to your eyes. With the middle finger of each hand at the bridge of your nose, make two circles up and over each eyebrow and under each eye, applying gentle pressure as you do so. Repeat as often as you like.
With your thumbs and index fingers, pinch several times along your eyebrows from the inner to outer ends.

Hold the pinch at the innermost edge of the brows to ease a tension headache.

Complete the massage by tapping your face with your fingertips from chin to forehead, forehead to chin. Give yourself a few minutes to enjoy the immediate sensation of relief. Eyes closed, gently cup your cheeks in your hands. Then, to further relax the muscles and dispel your inner tensions, smile.

Self-massagers who aren't contortionists should do some simple stretches to relax their back muscles. Stretch your arms behind your head as far as you can. Simultaneously, point your toes and stretch your legs. Hold that stretch from your fingertips to the tips of your toes for a count of 30. Release. Repeat. Five repeats or so should have a beneficial effect on those stress-kinks which have invaded your back muscles.

COLOR THERAPY

What color is your stress? Imagine your stress vibrating around you, then try to see what color it is. Is it red? Orange? A sharp chartreuse? Perhaps it is black?

If you can't visualize it, what color would you guess your stress to be?

Now conjure in your mind's eye any color which symbolizes tranquillity for you. Maybe a blue, the color of sea and sky. Or perhaps the green of trees, fields and gardens.

Visualize again the stress color, now send it away. Some people find it helps to brush a hand across their face from one side to the other in a wiping-away gesture, or to shake their hands flipping the stress color out from the fingertips.

In its place, let the color of your calm flow in to fill your consciousness. Slightly cupping your hands and very slowly and very lightly brushing them over your face, head and neck does seem to enhance the process. Besides, this sensual touch reminds you of how pleasant a relaxed body can feel.

BREATHING

Anytime, anywhere, you can slow yourself down, retrieve your sense of what's fundamentally important in your life by taking a slow deep breath. Then another. And another.

Deep breathe with your eyes closed. Do it when you wake in the morning rigid with tension, and again in the shower. Breathe deeply during your lunch hour and while you're waiting on the telephone. Breathe in silence or with music. And certainly do some deep even breaths before you go into that meeting or before you tell your children or your partner for the umpteenth time to put their dirty laundry in the basket, the lid down on the lavatory, the milk in the refrigerator or to feed the dog. When your head hits the pillow at night, do gentle deep breathing, and with each exhalation consciously make your heart beat slow down to match your breathing.

*The freeway is ... the place where they
(Angelenos) spend the two calmest and most
rewarding hours of their daily lives.*

Reyner Banham —

Los Angeles: the Architecture of Four Ecologies

*Reinforce the effect of deep breathing with vaporized essential oils let
loose in a quiet room. There is no need to restrict yourself to your home
territory. Who would know or care if at lunchtime you closed your door
and converted your office into a temporary haven, scented with your
chosen aromatic fragrance? Breathe deeply and regularly through
the nostrils — breathe in tranquillity and blow out stress.*

*For maximum effect, lie on the floor, arms a few inches to the sides
of your body, palms facing upwards. If you wish, use pillows to make
yourself more comfortable. Try one tucked under your neck, another
behind your knees to take any pressure off your lower back. Toss a
comforting rug over yourself. Close your eyes and breathe in, deeply,
through your nose. Hold for a few seconds. Breathe out, slowly,
also through your nose. Allow a few seconds to pass before
inhaling again. Repeat three times or more if you like.*

MEDITATING

Imagine your mind having rooms for special functions. Declare one of these a stress-free sector where "busy", "responsibility" and "hurry" are bad words. You can create other rooms which will serve these aspects of your life very well at the proper time and in the right place. Your stress-free mental space is a place of retreat for you and you alone.

It works especially well if you can give yourself 10 to 20 minutes at a set time each day to visit this room, to allow yourself to experience simply being.

Tempting, isn't it? And so easy.
Begin by seating yourself comfortably.
Close your eyes and concentrate on something of your choice.

You might like to imagine a rural scene at dawn, a city skyline at dusk. You might prefer to concentrate aurally, repeating a single word that appeals to you or listening to music. Becoming conscious of the sounds from nature is at once uplifting and soothing. Even the hum of traffic in the distance can induce feelings of deep relaxation.

YOU MIGHT PREFER TO KEEP YOUR EYES OPEN AND GAZE AT SOME PARTICULAR OBJECT IN NATURE SUCH AS ONE LEAF OR BLADE OF GRASS. MERGE YOURSELF WITH IT AS PART OF THE NATURAL WORLD AND SHARE ITS HARMONIES.

GENTLY REFOCUS YOUR ATTENTION AS THOUGHTS AND FEELINGS TUG IT THIS WAY AND THAT. GRADUALLY YOU'LL BECOME AWARE OF A SENSE OF INNER STILLNESS.

YOU CAN MEDITATE AS OFTEN AS YOU LIKE THROUGHOUT THE DAY — DURING MORNING AND AFTERNOON COFFEE BREAKS, BEFORE AND AFTER MEETINGS, ON THE 8:05 AM MONDAY TO FRIDAY COMMUTER SPECIAL, IN AIRPORT LOUNGES.

TO MAKE THE MOST OF MEDITATING TO RELIEVE STRESS, AS SOON AS YOU'VE EASED YOURSELF BACK INTO AN ALERT STATE, NOTE ANYTHING SIGNIFICANT WHICH FLOATED INTO YOUR MIND.

YOU MAY FIND THAT SOLUTIONS TO PARTICULARLY BOTHERSOME PROBLEMS WILL COME TO YOU DURING THESE MEDITATION SESSIONS. MANY CREATIVE PEOPLE FIND THEIR MOST BRILLIANT IDEAS AND SOLUTIONS TO CREATIVE PROBLEMS COME TO THEM IN MEDITATIVE MOMENTS — LET THE UNCONSCIOUS WORK IT OUT, THEY SAY.

AT BEDTIME, TAKE A FEW MINUTES TO REVIEW WHAT NOTIONS CAME TO YOU DURING YOUR MEDITATION AND HOW AND WHEN YOU IMPLEMENTED OR SHOULD IMPLEMENT THEM.

AT FIRST, YOU MIGHT FIND YOU DON'T DO ANYTHING WITH THE INFORMATION EMERGING DURING MEDITATION, BUT AFTER A WHILE YOU'LL NOTICE THAT YOU ARE MAKING CHANGES FOR THE BETTER IN YOUR LIFE, THAT YOU'RE HANDLING EVERYTHING JUST THAT BIT BETTER AT HOME, AT WORK AND AT PLAY. YOU'LL NOTICE THAT YOU NO LONGER FIND LIFE AS STRESSFUL AS YOU ONCE DID.

> *Nothing in the affairs of men is*
> *worthy of great anxiety.*
>
> Plato — *Republic*

A TOP-TO-TOE

STRESS DE-BRIEF

STRUNG-OUT TO SNAPPING POINT?

GET OUT YOUR ESSENTIAL OIL, YOUR ROOM VAPORIZER, HAVE YOUR AROMATIC BATH, YOUR MASSAGE, GRAB YOUR PILLOWS AND YOUR COMFORTER, SET YOURSELF IN POSITION AND BREATHE DEEPLY. WHEN YOU EXHALE FOR THE THIRD TIME, DO SO THROUGH YOUR MOUTH AS THOUGH YOU WERE SIGHING. YOUR STRESS DE-BRIEFING HAS BEGUN.

CONTINUE TO FOCUS ON YOUR BREATHING BUT BROADEN YOUR FOCUS TO INCLUDE YOUR FEET. INHALE THROUGH YOUR NOSE, AND COUNT TO FOUR WHILE CURLING AND UNCURLING YOUR TOES. RELAX YOUR FEET AS YOU BREATHE OUT, AGAIN THROUGH YOUR MOUTH.

inhale

Follow this inhale-flex and exhale-relax process next to your calves, then knees, thighs, buttocks, abdomen, chest, back, hands, arms, shoulders, neck, head and face and feel that stress release.

Take a few deep breaths and then mentally sweep your body from top to toe. Your mind is on a search and destroy mission for pockets of lingering stress. Treat remnants of tension in any spot with supplementary doses of the de-brief technique.

When you complete the scan and streamline stage, simply stay where you are, **DOING NOTHING**, breathing normally — that is, quietly and gently as though it were second nature to you — which it is.

exhale

AFTER AT LEAST FIVE MINUTES, BUT MORE IF YOU CAN, PUT YOUR HANDS BEHIND YOUR HEAD, REACHING AS FAR AS YOU CAN IN THAT DIRECTION WITH YOUR FINGERTIPS AND IN THE OTHER WITH YOUR POINTED TOES.

THEN SLOWLY CURL YOURSELF INTO A SITTING POSITION AND SLOWLY RISE TO YOUR KNEES, THEN TO YOUR FEET. ONE MORE BIG STRETCH, ARMS OVERHEAD AND THEN BROUGHT GENTLY DOWN BESIDE YOUR BODY AND SLIGHTLY TO THE BACK. MAKE A FEW CIRCLES WITH YOUR SHOULDERS, FIRST ONE WAY, THEN THE OTHER. SHRUG SLOWLY. AND AGAIN.

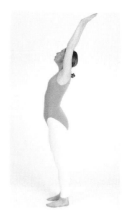

Here lies a poor woman who always was tired,
For she lived in a place where help wasn't hired.
Her last words on earth were, Dear friends I am going
Where washing ain't done nor sweeping nor sewing,
And everything there is exact to my wishes,
For there they don't eat and there's no washing of dishes ....
Don't mourn for me now, don't mourn for me never,
For I'm going to do nothing for ever and ever.

Anon — Epitaph

STRESS AND YOUR WEIGHT

STRESS AND SKINNY OFTEN GO TOGETHER. YOU GET TOO BUSY TO EAT OR ELSE STRESS SEEMS TO KICK YOUR METABOLISM INTO TOP GEAR AND YOU BURN UP EVERYTHING YOU SWALLOW. BUT THEN STRESS AND SUPERFLUOUS POUNDS AND INCHES FREQUENTLY MAKE INSEPARABLE PARTNERS, TOO. YOU GORGE ON FATTENING COMFORT FOOD AND GIVE UP EXERCISING BECAUSE YOU HAVE "TOO MUCH TO DO" OR ARE "TOO TIRED".

ACCORDING TO SOME RESEARCH FROM YALE UNIVERSITY WOMEN WITH RUNAWAY STRESS HAVE THICKER WAISTLINES AND FATTER TUMMIES THAN THOSE WHO PRACTICE GOOD STRESS MANAGEMENT. STRESS ACTIVATES THE BODY'S PRODUCTION OF THE HORMONE CORTISOL. EXCESS STRESS EQUALS EXCESS CORTISOL. THIS HORMONE DIRECTS BODY FAT TO THE BODY-FRONT, LOCATION OF THE FAST-FUEL DEPOT FOR THE FIGHT OR FLIGHT STRESS RESPONSES.

Get Away From It All

It was Einstein who made the real trouble.
He announced in 1905 that there was no such
thing as absolute rest. After that there never was.

Stephen Leacock — *The Boy I Left Behind Me*

Take a holiday.

Go to a health retreat. It will offer you
a few days of amazing contrast to
your current, stressful lifestyle.

A Weekend Away At Home

Consider the merits of a weekend at your very own health resort.

Imagine ... Friday night spent doing some or all of those wonderfully de-stressing things you can do with essential oils or fragrant herbs. Go to bed as late as you like. You don't have to get up at any particular time in the morning.

When you do get out of bed on Saturday, have a glass of juice before a session of meditation or some deep breathing and body stretching.

THEN HAVE BREAKFAST. KEEP IT HEALTHY, AND LIGHT. NO HEAPED PLATTERS OF EGGS, SAUSAGES AND BACON.

WHILE WAITING AT LEAST AN HOUR FOR YOUR DIGESTIVE SYSTEM TO DO ITS WORK, READ THE PAPERS, LISTEN TO MUSIC OR JUST POTTER.

THEN PULL ON SOME COMFY CLOTHES, HAVE A DRINK OF WATER AND TAKE A BRISK WALK FOR 30 TO 45 MINUTES.

DRINK SOME MORE WATER WHEN YOU COME HOME AND HAVE A HEALTHY SNACK IF YOU'RE FEELING PECKISH. AN APPLE, A BANANA, A COUPLE OF PLAIN CRACKERS WOULD BE SUITABLE.

DO SOME MORE STRETCHES AND DEEP BREATHING BEFORE GETTING INTO AN AROMATIC SHOWER OR BATH.

MAKE THIS A BEAUTY SESSION AS WELL. HAVE A FACIAL. HAVE A BODY SCRUB. TAKE TIME OUT FOR A HAIR-CONDITIONING TREATMENT. GIVE YOURSELF A PEDICURE AND MANICURE, SAVING THE FINAL, POLISHING TOUCHES FOR LATER. WHILE YOU LUXURIATE IN THE TUB, SIP A HEALTHY, RELAXING HERBAL TEA OR SOME FRUIT OR VEGETABLE JUICE.

HAVING HAULED YOURSELF RELUCTANTLY FROM THOSE FRAGRANT WATERS, TRY A STRESS DE-BRIEF, FLEXING AND RELAXING YOUR MUSCLES FROM ONE END OF YOUR BODY TO THE OTHER.

LUNCH IS GOING TO BE YOUR MAIN MEAL OF THE DAY BUT THAT DOESN'T MEAN OVERLOADING YOUR SYSTEM. STICK TO A SMALL TO MEDIUM PORTION OF LEAN MEAT, CHICKEN OR FISH WITH VEGETABLES OR SALAD. IF YOU'RE HUNGRY, FILL UP WITH MORE VEGETABLES, WHOLEMEAL OR GRAIN BREAD OR FRESH FRUIT.

WHILE YOU'RE DIGESTING LUNCH, TAKE A LIGHT NAP IF YOU LIKE.

THEN GO FOR ANOTHER WALK, RUN, BICYCLE RIDE OR SWIM.

TAKE ANOTHER BATH OR SHOWER WITH THE AROMATIC OILS AND FOLLOW WITH SESSIONS OF DEEP-BREATHING, STRETCHING AND MASSAGE.

READ, LISTEN TO MUSIC OR MEDITATE BEFORE DINNER.

KEEP DINNER LIGHT BUT NUTRITIOUS. AN OMELETTE, PERHAPS. A SMALL BOWL OF PASTA WITH YOUR FAVORITE SAUCE. FOR SEAFOOD LOVERS, OYSTERS OR PRAWNS OR BOTH. A SALAD. A SLICE OR TWO OF FRESH BREAD OR TOAST (EASY ON THE BUTTER). FRUIT JUICE. HERBAL TEA.

IF YOU'RE DESPERATELY MISSING YOUR TEA OR COFFEE, WHISKY OR WINE, THEN HAVE SOME. THERE'S NO POINT IN BEING BRUTAL WITH YOURSELF. THAT'S NOT WHAT THIS WEEKEND IS ABOUT. IT'S ABOUT BEING GOOD TO YOURSELF. BUT DO TAKE IT EASY WITH THE CAFFEINE AND ALCOHOL. TOO MUCH AND YOU'LL DEFEAT YOUR DE-STRESS PURPOSE.

AFTER DINNER, READ, MAYBE WATCH AN AMUSING VIDEO OR TELEVISION SHOW (NOTHING HEAVY, THOUGH), CATCH A CONCERT ON YOUR RADIO. GO FOR A STROLL AROUND YOUR BLOCK. SIT AT YOUR WINDOW OR BALCONY IF YOU HAVE ONE AND GAZE AT THE NIGHT SKY. BY NOW YOU MIGHT BE REALLY HOOKED ON AROMATIC BATHS AS RELAXANTS. YOU WON'T SHRINK IF YOU HAVE YET ANOTHER BEFORE GOING TO BED.

SUNDAY, REPEAT THE KIND OF DAY YOU GAVE YOURSELF ON SATURDAY, USING THE SAME INGREDIENTS BUT MIXING THEM TO SUIT YOURSELF.

MONDAY MORNING, YOU WON'T KNOW YOURSELF. PLAN TO GIVE YOURSELF THAT LITTLE EXTRA TIME YOU NEED AT LEAST TO DO SOME DEEP BREATHING AND BODY STRETCHING BUT PREFERABLY TO TAKE A BRISK WALK FOR HALF AN HOUR BEFORE YOU LAUNCH INTO YOUR WORKING WEEK.

QUICK CALMERS

SAY "NO"

WALK – MARCH UP AND DOWN ON THE SPOT FOR A FEW MINUTES.

DANCE – WITH OR WITHOUT MUSIC. SING AS YOU MOVE. IN FRONT OF THE MIRROR OR ROUND THE ROOM. BOOGIE. SWIRL. WALTZ. TAP. HULA. TANGO.

PLAY – BROWSE IN YOUR BOOKSHOP OR MUSIC STORE, YOUR PERFUMERY. GO SHOPPING FOR SOME ANTI-STRESS TOYS: A DARTBOARD, A PUNCHING BAG OR CUSHION, A SLAM-DUNK KIT TO INSTAL IN YOUR OFFICE, A YO-YO, A RUBBER BALL TO SQUEEZE AWAY YOUR TENSION, WORRY BEADS.

Don't panic

Douglas Adams —
The hitchhiker's guide to the galaxy

Goodness never means simply acceding to everyone else's idea of what you ought to be doing (for them). Adult virtue includes being able to decide what you can do, in terms of the importance you assign a task and the cost to you of performing it.

Judith Martin — *Miss Manners' Guide to Rearing Perfect Children*

I'm Burlington Bertie
I rise at ten thirty and saunter along like a toff,
I walk down the Strand with my gloves on my hand,
Then I walk down again with them off.

W.F. Hargreaves — *Burlington Bertie from Bow*

GO SLOW – WHEN YOU WALK, SLOW YOURSELF TO A MEASURED STRIDE. SLOW DOWN YOUR SPEECH, MAKING YOURSELF SOUND SUPER-RELAXED. EAT SLOWLY. SAY THE WORD "SLOW" ALOUD OR TO YOURSELF. AND SAY IT SLOWLY.

TAKE A WHOLE HOUR FOR LUNCH

I suspect guys who say, "I just send out for a sandwich for lunch" as lazy men trying to impress me.

Jimmy Cannon — *Nobody Asked Me, But ...*
(New York Post)

Brother, do you know a nicer occupation,
Matter of fact, neither do I,
Than standing on the corner
Watching all the girls go by?

Frank Loesser — *Standing on the Corner*

INSTANT REPLAYS – *defuse your stress with a flashback. Review the past few hours, the past day, the past week. Edit all the bad things. Zoom in for a close-up of all the good things that happened to you and the good things that you did, your achievements, your kindnesses. Praise yourself. Thank yourself.*

COPYCATTING — *think of someone you know or some public figure, some character in a novel or film, who possesses calm. Copy their calm. Absorb their calm. Make it your own.*

SELF-CENTER – WHAT IS IT THAT IS DRIVING YOU CRAZY RIGHT NOW? NOT UNDERLYING, LONG-STANDING IRRITANTS, BUT WHATEVER IS GETTING ON YOUR NERVES THIS VERY MINUTE.

Pooh began to feel a little more comfortable, because when you are a Bear of Very Little Brain, and you Think of Things, you find sometimes that a Thing which seemed very Thingish inside you is quite different when it gets out into the open and has other people looking at it.

A.A. Milne — *The House at Pooh Corner*

DON'T JUST KNOW THE ANSWER. SAY IT. SILENTLY. THE FINAL STEP IS TO CONSCIOUSLY AND DELIBERATELY CONCENTRATE ON YOUR BREATHING. SLOWING IT JUST A FRACTION WILL GIVE YOU THE EDGE ON YOUR STRESS.

MINI BODY-WORK TECHNIQUES

The feet

Slip off your left shoe, cross your left leg over your right, clench your right hand into a fist. Inhale through your nose. Exhale through either nose or mouth but as you do so press your fist into the acupressure point within the hollow of your left foot, beneath the arch. Release and repeat the pressure as many times as you like, adjusting the pressure to suit your comfort zone. Repeat for the right foot.

The face

Scrunch your face up. Relax. Raise your eyebrows and then lower them. Open your eyes as widely as you can and then let them relax. Close your eyes. Wriggle your nose. Tug gently at your ear lobes. Smile a big smile. Give a big yawn. Hands to shoulders, squeeze and release the big muscles from shoulder tip to neck. Rub the back of your neck. Pat yourself all over: forehead, eyes, sides of nose, cheeks, chin, neck, shoulders and upper chest.

The wrists

HOLD YOUR LEFT WRIST SO THAT THE PALM OF YOUR HAND FACES UPWARDS. WITH THE MIDDLE FINGER OF YOUR RIGHT HAND, TRACE AN IMAGINARY LINE DOWN FROM THE MIDDLE FINGER OF YOUR LEFT HAND TO AN ACUPRESSURE POINT APPROXIMATELY $1\frac{1}{2}$ INCHES (3 CM) FROM THE EDGE OF YOUR PALM. INHALE THROUGH YOUR NOSE. EXHALE THROUGH EITHER YOUR NOSE OR YOUR MOUTH, BUT AS YOU EXHALE PRESS YOUR DOWN AS HARD AS YOU CAN BEAR ON THAT PRESSURE POINT.

Stand tall

SLOWLY RAISE YOUR ARMS ABOUT YOUR HEAD. STRETCH. INHALE AND HOLD THE STRETCH FOR A COUNT OF 10. EXHALE AND LOWER YOUR ARMS. REPEAT TO SUIT YOURSELF.

YOUR LIFE TRANSFORMED

By now you will probably realize that most of your stress is not only unnecessary but is robbing your life of pleasure. When you find yourself under stress, ask: Will your life be ruined as a result of this situation? Will anyone else's?

If the answer is yes, then some appropriate action — not worrying inaction — must be taken. If the answer is no, then your suffering is out of proportion to the issue, and you are probably ruining all that could be good during this time.

Life presents difficulties — perhaps you might now prefer to call them challenges. If something can be changed, change it. If it can't, step back and let the situation ride itself out.

So, whenever your heart beats faster, your breath becomes shallow, and your muscles rigid, ask yourself just how important is this thing in the scheme of your life, breathe deeply, then deal with the matter appropriately.

If you take to heart this simple philosophy and practice the hints for stress relief presented in this book, difficulties will dissolve as though by magic, and a daily sense of joy will be yours once more

Published by Lansdowne Publishing Pty Ltd
Sydney, Australia
First published in 1996
© Copyright: Lansdowne Publishing Pty Ltd
Chief Executive Publisher: Jane Curry
Publishing Manager: Deborah Nixon
Production Manager: Sally Stokes
Project Co-ordinator: Jenny Coren
Designer: Sylvie Abecassis
Cover design concept: Liz Seymour
Set in Cochin on QuarkXpress
Printed in Hong Kong
Produced by Mandarin Offset
Cataloguing-in-Publication data has been lodged
at the National Library of Australia
ISBN 1 86302 497 2